# ANATOMY
# COLORING BOOK

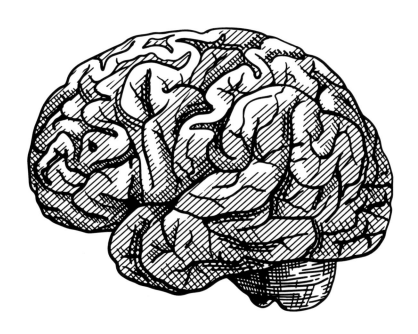

## Anatomy Unlocked

# 1 CONTENTS

# Discovering Human Body

Hello and welcome to our anatomy coloring book! Through colorable graphics and extensive text, this book provides a novel and engaging approach to learning about the human anatomy.

The book's first portion presents an overview of the human body and its many systems. You will investigate the respiratory, digestive, circulatory, and other systems, obtaining a thorough grasp of how each system contributes to our overall health.

The second half of the book concentrates on the skeletal system, which serves as our bodies' framework. You'll learn about the numerous types of bones and their functions, as well as the various joints that allow us to move and accomplish various jobs.

The book's third and final portion looks into the muscular system, which collaborates with the skeletal system to allow us to move and perform a range of jobs. You will learn about the numerous types of muscle tissue, the mechanics of muscle movement, and the significance of correct muscle maintenance and care.

You will have the option to color and name comprehensive drawings of the human anatomy throughout the book, confirming your grasp of the principles provided. Whether you are a student, a healthcare professional, or simply someone curious in their own body, this book provides a fun and engaging approach to learn about the mysteries of human anatomy. So take your pencils and prepare to be enthralled by the intriguing world of the human body!

# How to use

- Gather your supplies: Before you start coloring, make sure you have everything you need, such as colored pencils, markers, or crayons, as well as a sharpener and eraser.

- Select your colors: Choose the colors you wish to use and organize them. To keep track of which colors belong to various structures, a color code or legend may be useful.

- Begin with light colors: Begin by coloring in the image's lighter sections. This allows you to gradually build up the color and avoid coloring over key structures.

- When coloring, use a delicate touch to avoid smearing the image by pushing too hard. This will help to maintain the image's lines and details crisp and distinct.

- Color in pieces: Divide the image into smaller sections and color each one individually. This will assist you in staying organized and avoiding coloring over incorrect structures.

- Take note of labels and descriptions: As you color, take note of the labels and descriptions of the structures. These will assist you in understanding the functioning and relationships of various body parts.

By following these guidelines, you will be able to color correctly the illustrations and gain a better knowledge of the intricate components and systems that comprise the human body. Have a good time!

# 2 INTRODUCTION TO THE HUMAN BODY

## 2.1 THE ANATOMY FIELD

Anatomy is a field of biology and medicine that studies and describes the anatomy of living creatures. Human anatomy, animal anatomy (zootomy), and plant anatomy (phytology) are all covered. Anatomy has been studied for nearly 2,000 years, beginning with the Ancient Greeks. Human anatomy, in particular, focuses on the human body's structures and functions. Understanding anatomy is essential for practicing medicine and other health-related areas.

The word "anatomy" comes from the Greek terms "ana," which means "up," and "tome," which means "cutting." Anatomical studies have traditionally required dissecting creatures to understand their interior structures. However, developments in imaging technology have made it feasible to examine the inner workings of the body without dissection.

Anatomy may be studied in two ways: microscopic anatomy and gross, or macroscopic, anatomy. Microscopic anatomy studies the architecture of cells and tissues using microscopes, whereas gross anatomy studies the structures of organs and systems apparent to the human eye.

### 2.1.1 Gross anatomy

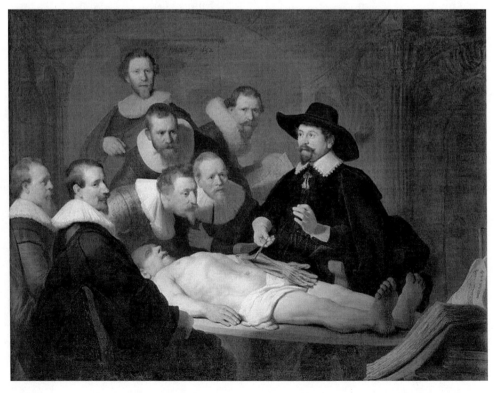

*Rembrandt - The Anatomy Lesson of Dr Nicolaes Tulp Wikimedia*

Gross or macroscopic anatomy is a discipline of medicine that studies biological features visible to the naked eye. Both invasive and noninvasive approaches can be used to study this sort of anatomy.

Dissection is a typical way of studying gross anatomy that involves scientists cutting apart an organism and inspecting its interior parts. Endoscopy is another diagnostic and research technique that involves inserting a long, thin tube with a camera at the end into various regions of the body for evaluation.

Injecting opaque dyes into blood arteries and employing imaging equipment such as angiography to see how the circulatory system works are less intrusive means of studying gross anatomy. MRI scans, CT scans, PET scans, X-rays, and ultrasounds are also used to examine the inside anatomy of live creatures.

Medical and dentistry students may also do dissection as part of their practical work during their education, utilizing human corpses to understand gross anatomy. Overall, gross anatomy gives vital insights into the greater architecture of organs and organ systems, and it is critical for understanding how the human body works.

### 2.1.2 Human body systems

Gross anatomy students often learn about the primary organ systems of the human body. The human body contains 11 organ systems, each with its unique structure and function, each of the following systems collaborates to keep the body's general health and function in check, and a detailed understanding of their structure, and function is essential for both healthcare practitioners and researchers:

| Organ System | Main Functions |
|---|---|
| Skeletal system | Through the utilization of bones, cartilage, and ligaments, it provides support, protection, and mobility. |
| Muscular system | Through the use of muscles and tendons, it allows mobility and sustains the body's posture. |
| Lymphatic system | Produces and transports white blood cells and lymphatic fluid, which aids the body's defense against infections and illnesses. |
| Respiratory system | Through breathing, it facilitates the exchange of gases (oxygen and carbon dioxide) between the body and the environment. |
| Digestive system | Food is processed and nutrients are extracted through the mouth, esophagus, stomach, intestines, and other organs. |
| Nervous system | Controls and coordinates the functioning of the body via the brain, spinal cord, and nerves. |
| Endocrine system | Regulates hormone synthesis and metabolism by using organs such as the thyroid, pancreas, and adrenal glands. |
| Cardiovascular system | Blood circulates throughout the body, supplying oxygen and nutrients to cells and eliminating waste via the heart and blood arteries. |
| Urinary system | Using the kidneys, bladder, and urethra, it removes waste from the body and helps control blood pressure and electrolyte levels. |
| Reproductive system | Allows for the generation of children by using the male and female reproductive organs. |
| Integumentary system | Through the use of skin, hair, and nails, it protects the body from environmental harm and helps regulate body temperature. |

## 2.1.3  Microscopic anatomy

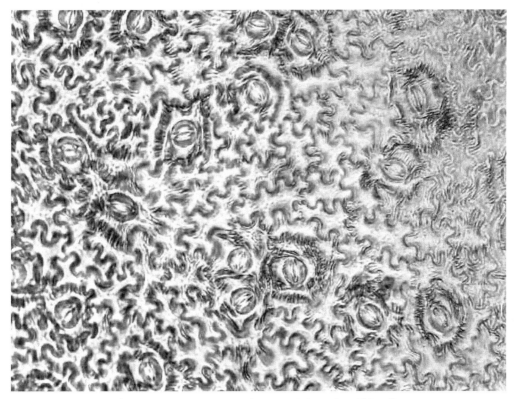

*lant anatomy microscopic shots- Fatsia japonica Wikimedia*

Microscopic anatomy, often known as histology, is the study of cells and tissues that are too tiny to be seen with the naked eye in animals, humans, and plants. Histology allows researchers to learn about the structure and function of cells, as well as how they interact with one another.

Sectioning and staining are common histology processes for examining tissues and cells. Sectioning is the technique of cutting tissues into thin slices for detailed examination, whereas staining is the process of adding or intensifying color to help identify specific tissues under investigation. Electron and light microscopes can be used to analyze tissues and cells.

Biology, veterinary medicine, medicine, and other areas of life science all benefit from an understanding of histology. Under a microscope, for example, tissue inspection can reveal the existence of malignant cells and assist researchers in learning how they behave and damage healthy tissue. Histology is a useful technique for studying live creatures and their underlying structures.

Histology has a variety of essential applications, including:

1. **Teaching**: To help students understand the microstructures of biological tissues, histology slides are utilized in teaching labs.

2. **Diagnosis**: Doctors may extract tissue samples or biopsies from patients with suspected cancer or other disorders, which are subsequently evaluated in a lab by a histologist.
3. **Forensic investigations**: In unexpected or questionable circumstances, histological study of certain biological tissues can assist forensic professionals in determining the cause of death.
4. **Autopsies**: Histological analysis is also utilized in postmortem investigations of deceased individuals and animals to determine the reasons of death.
5. **Archeology**: Biological samples from archeological sites can give important information on ancient societies' habits, diets, and illnesses.

In general, histology is a flexible tool that aids in research, medicine, and other professions by providing insights into the microstructures and functions of live creatures.


## 2.1.4   Histopathology

Histology laboratories include histotechnicians, histotechnologists, and histology technicians who are in charge of processing biological tissue samples for examination. Histopathologists, often known as pathologists, are doctors who study and evaluate samples.

Histology technicians may process tissue samples from patients seeking a diagnosis, suspects in a forensic inquiry, or deceased persons. Trimming and conserving the samples, replacing water with paraffin wax, slicing the tissue thinly, mounting it on slides, and applying stains to make specific areas visible are all part of the procedure.

After the samples are produced, a histopathologist studies and analyses the cells and tissues. Other healthcare providers can utilize the histopathologist's findings to choose the best course of therapy for patients or to aid in forensic investigations to ascertain the cause of death.

Individuals in the United States must be certified by the American Society for Clinical Pathology in order to work as a histotechnologist. They can do so by finishing a degree program that involves math, biology, and chemistry as well as acquiring on-the-job experience, or by enrolling in an authorized histology school. Higher education is also accessible in this sector.

Individuals normally need to finish a four-year medical degree program, followed by three to seven years of internship and residency programs, to become a pathologist.

## 2.1.5 Studying anatomy

Many healthcare professions, such as paramedics, nurses, physical therapists, occupational therapists, medical physicians, prosthetists, and biological scientists, need a thorough grasp of gross anatomy and histology to do their responsibilities successfully.

The study of structures visible to the human eye, such as organs, bones, and muscles, is referred to as gross anatomy. Histology, on the other hand, is the microscopic examination of tissues and cells.

For example, a paramedic may need to swiftly locate a vein in order to provide medicine or set up an IV line. To monitor vital signs and spot any anomalies, nurses may need to grasp the architecture of a patient's circulatory system. To build rehabilitation strategies, physical therapists and occupational therapists may need to identify specific muscles and bones. To effectively diagnose and treat patients, medical physicians must have a good grasp of anatomy. To develop and install prosthetic devices, prosthetists must grasp the anatomy of limbs and joints. Biological scientists examine the structure and function of living creatures using anatomical knowledge.

In the end, many healthcare workers and scientists require a thorough grasp of anatomy and histology in order to deliver effective treatment and improve their areas.

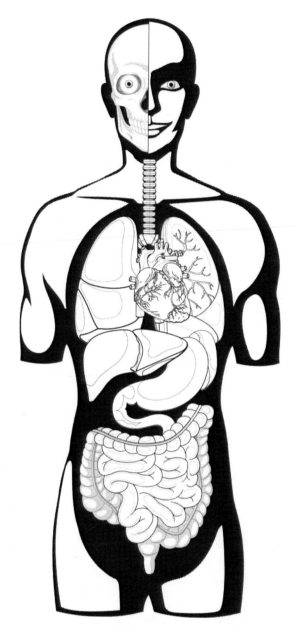

*Human anatomy model with different systems - Free Pic*

The human body is a sophisticated creature with a well-organized structure. It is composed of many systems, organs, tissues, and cells that collaborate to conduct important processes required for living. In this chapter, we will look at how the human body is organized and how its many components interact together.

The human body is organized into multiple layers, beginning with the smallest unit of life, the cell. Cells are the fundamental building elements of all living species, and humans have several cell types that perform distinct activities. These cells create tissues, which are clusters of cells that collaborate to accomplish a certain purpose.

In the human body, there are four kinds of tissues: epithelial, connective, muscular, and nerve tissue. Connective tissue supports and links different areas of the body, whereas epithelial tissue covers and lines the body's surfaces and cavities. Muscle tissue is in charge of movement, whereas nerve tissue is in charge of communication and coordination between different areas of the body.

### 2.2.1 Cells

Cells are the fundamental building components of all living entities, including humans. They are the tiniest unit of life, performing all of the processes required for an organism to exist.

In the human body, there are many distinct types of cells, each with a unique role. Muscle cells, for example, contract and allow movement, nerve cells send information throughout the body, and red blood cells provide oxygen to the body's tissues.

A cell membrane surrounds the cell and controls what enters and leaves the cell. A nucleus includes the genetic material of the cell, as well as organelles such as mitochondria, which provide energy, and the endoplasmic reticulum, which is involved in protein synthesis.

Cells can divide and duplicate themselves, which is required for tissue and organ development, repair, and maintenance. Cells, on the other hand, can become damaged or sick, leading to disorders such as cancer.

Understanding cell structure and function is critical for healthcare professionals and scientists diagnosing and treating a wide range of illnesses and ailments. Cell research advances have resulted in the creation of new medicines and therapies for a variety of ailments, including cancer and genetic abnormalities.

### 2.2.2 Tissues

Tissues are collections of related cells that collaborate to execute a certain purpose. In the human body, there are four kinds of tissues: epithelial, connective, muscular, and nerve tissue.

Epithelial tissue covers and lines the body's surfaces and cavities, acting as a protective barrier. It can be present in the skin, digestive tract lining, and respiratory system.

Connective tissue links and supports various bodily components. It consists of bone, cartilage, blood vessels, adipose tissue (fat), and fibrous tissue.

Muscle tissue, which is found in the skeletal, smooth, and cardiac muscles, is responsible for movement. Smooth muscle is present in organs such as the digestive tract and blood vessels and is responsible for involuntary movement. Skeletal muscle is related to bones and allows voluntary movement. Cardiac muscle is situated in the heart and is in charge of pumping blood around the body.

Nervous tissue is in charge of communication and coordination between various areas of the body. It consists of neurons (specialized cells that send electrical impulses) and glial cells (support and protect neurons).

Cancer can form as a result of abnormal cell development and division, and some connective tissue problems can affect the body's tissue durability and stability, thus understanding the many types of tissues and their roles is essential for successfully diagnosing and treating a broad range of ailments.

### 2.2.3    Organs

Organs are structures composed of two or more types of tissues that collaborate to carry out a given function. Many organs in the human body perform various roles.

The heart, for example, is an organ composed of muscle and connective tissue. Its primary job is to circulate blood throughout the body. Another example of an organ is the lungs, which are made up of epithelial tissue, muscular tissue, and connective tissue and are in charge of gas exchange between the body and the environment.

The liver is a multifunctional organ that filters toxic compounds from the blood, produces bile to aid in fat digestion, and stores glucose for energy. It is made up of three types of tissue: connective tissue, epithelial tissue, and nerve tissue.

Another crucial organ is the brain, which is made up of nerve tissue and is in charge of coordinating and managing the body's processes as well as processing information from the environment.

Each organ has a distinct purpose and collaborates with other organs and tissues to keep the body running smoothly. Understanding the anatomy and function of organs is critical for healthcare professionals diagnosing and treating illnesses and ailments that affect them. Liver illness, for example, can impair the organ's capacity to filter poisons from the blood, whereas brain diseases can impair cognitive function and behavior.

### 2.2.4    Systems

A system in anatomy is a set of organs that work together to provide a certain function in the body. The human body includes multiple interrelated systems that work together to sustain general health and function.

The circulatory system is in charge of moving oxygen, nutrients, and waste throughout the body. It consists of the heart, blood arteries, and blood itself, and it guarantees that all cells receive the oxygen and nutrients they require to operate correctly.

The respiratory system is in charge of absorbing oxygen and expending carbon dioxide. It consists of the lungs, trachea, and bronchi and keeps the body supplied with oxygen for cellular respiration.

The digestive system converts food into nutrients that the body can absorb. It is responsible for feeding the body with energy and nutrients for development and repair, and it includes the mouth, esophagus, stomach, intestines, liver, and pancreas.

To govern its operations, the nervous system coordinates and interacts with many sections of the body. It consists of the brain, spinal cord, and nerves and allows the body to detect and respond to environmental changes.

Hormones released by the endocrine system regulate various bodily functions, including development, metabolism, and reproduction. It is made up of glands such as the pituitary, thyroid, and adrenal glands.

The immune system defends the body against outside invaders such bacteria, viruses, and poisons. It consists of white blood cells, lymph nodes, and the spleen and aids in the prevention and treatment of infections.

The lymphatic system helps the body maintain fluid balance and combat infections. Lymph nodes, lymph arteries, and white blood cells are all part of it.

The urinary system excretes waste from the body. It consists of the kidneys, ureters, bladder, and urethra and is responsible for regulating the body's electrolyte balance.

The reproductive system, which comprises the testes, ovaries, uterus, and other reproductive organs, is in charge of reproduction.

The musculoskeletal system supports and structures the body while also allowing mobility. It consists of bones, muscles, and tendons.

The integumentary system protects the body from external harm and aids in temperature regulation. It consists of the skin, hair, and nails.

## 2.3   ANATOMICAL TERMINOLOGY

The terminology employed by anatomists and healthcare practitioners might be intimidating to individuals who are unfamiliar with it. The goal of this terminology, however, is not to confuse, but rather to enhance precision and eliminate medical mistakes. When defining the position of a scar, for example, using specific anatomical terminology avoids uncertainty. Anatomical terminologies are drawn from ancient Greek and Latin phrases that are no longer in common use, ensuring that their meanings stay consistent.

Anatomical terminology are made up of roots, prefixes, and suffixes that define organs, tissues, and situations in a brief and precise manner. The root of a phrase usually relates to a specific organ, tissue, or condition, but the prefix or suffix frequently gives extra information to characterize the root. The prefix "hyper-" in the phrase "hypertension" refers to "high" or "over," but the root "tension" alludes to pressure. As a result, the term "hypertension" refers to unusually high blood pressure.

## 2.3.1 Anatomical Position

To improve precision, anatomists standardize their technique to observing the body. The conventional body "map" or anatomical posture involves the body standing erect with feet shoulder-width apart and parallel, toes facing forward, much as maps are generally orientated with north at the top. As indicated in the figure, the upper limbs are extended out to each side, and the palms of the hands face front. Using this conventional posture reduces anatomical language misunderstanding. The phrases are used as though the body is in anatomical position, regardless of how it is positioned.

For example, a scar on the palm side of the wrist in the "anterior (front) carpal (wrist) region" would be present, and the term "anterior" would be used even if the hand was put palm down on a table. This standardized technique assures consistency in anatomical terminology regardless of the orientation of the body being described.

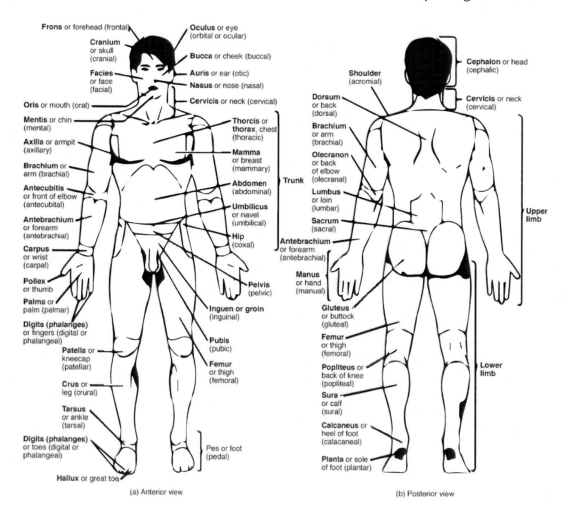

*OpenStax - Human Body Regions. Anatomical views of the human body are illustrated in (a) anterior and (b) posterior views. The body parts are labeled in boldface - Wikimedia Commons, CC BY SA 4.0 and CC BY 3.0*

The phrases "prone" and "supine" are used to describe the position of a laying body. The term "prone" refers to a face-down position, whereas "supine" refers to a face-up position. These phrases are especially relevant when defining the posture of the body during physical examinations or surgical operations when exact placement is required.

### 2.3.2 Regional Terms

The various parts of the human body have distinct words to improve accuracy, as seen in the figure. These phrases facilitate clear communication and assist to avoid misunderstandings.

For example, the term "brachium" refers to the upper arm, whereas "antebrachium" refers to the forearm rather than the less exact phrase "lower arm." Similarly, the term "femur" refers to the thigh, whereas "leg" or "crus" solely refers to the lower limb between the knee and ankle.

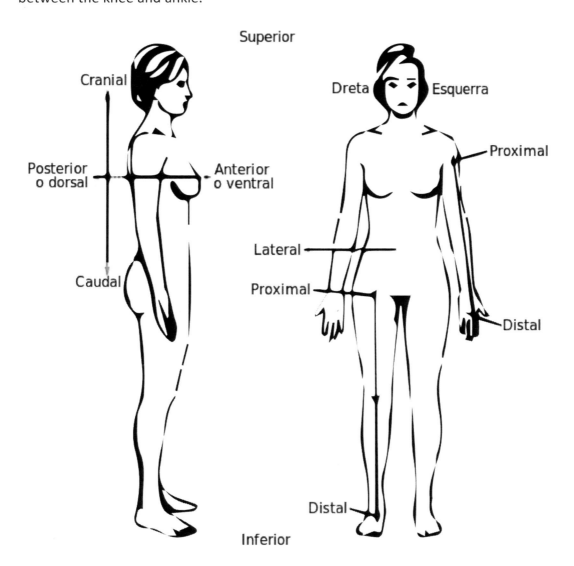

*OpenStax College/ Connexions - Human Body Directional Terminology. Paired directional words are depicted as they apply to the human body – Wikimedia Commons CC 3.0*

### 2.3.3   Directional Terms

Anatomy publications utilize directional terminology to explain the relative placements of various anatomical components. In the medical industry, these terminologies are critical for accurate communication. Understanding and memorizing these phrases might assist in avoiding misunderstanding while studying or discussing the locations of certain bodily parts.

- The term "**anterior**" (or "ventral") refers to the front or orientation of the body. The toes, for example, are located anterior to the foot.
- The term "**posterior**" (or "dorsal") refers to the back or the direction toward the back of the body. The popliteus muscle, for example, is located posterior to the patella.
- The term "**superior**" (or "cranial") refers to a place that is higher or higher than another region of the body. The orbits (eye sockets), for example, are superior than the oris (mouth).
- The term "**inferior**" (or "caudal") refers to a place below or lower than another region of the body, closer to the tail (the coccyx, or lowest part of the spinal column in humans). For example, the pelvis is lower than the abdomen.
- The term "**lateral**" refers to the side or direction of the body. The pollex (thumb) is lateral to the digits.
- The term "**medial**" refers to the center or orientation toward the center of the body. The medial toe is the hallux (large toe).
- The term "**proximal**" refers to a place in a limb that is closer to the site of attachment or the body's trunk. The brachium (upper arm) is proximal to the antebrachium (forearm), for example.
- "**Distal**" refers to a limb posture that is farther away from the site of attachment or the trunk of the body. The crus is located distal to the femur (thigh bone).
- The term "**superficial**" refers to a location closer to the body's surface. For example, the skin is just superficial to the bones.
- "**Deep**" refers to a place away from the body's surface. The brain is located deep within the skull.

### 2.3.4   Body Planes

In anatomy and medicine, a section is a two-dimensional surface of a three-dimensional structure that has been cut. Contrarily, the interpretation of body sections and scans depends on the viewer's understanding of the plane along which the section was formed. A plane is a two-dimensional imaginary surface that runs through the body, and there are three planes that are often used in anatomy and medicine. A vertical plane that separates the body or an organ into right and left sides is known as the sagittal plane. This plane is known as the midsagittal or median plane when it goes directly down the center of the body. It is referred to as a parasagittal plane or, less typically, a longitudinal plane if it splits the body into uneven right and left halves. The anterior (front) and posterior (rear) halves of the body or an organ are separated by the frontal plane. The frontal plane is also known as the coronal plane, from the Latin word "corona," which means "crown." The transverse plane is a plane that divides the body or organ into upper and lower halves horizontally. Cross-sections are pictures produced by transverse planes. Mastering these planes is essential for interpreting body scans and determining the position and orientation of various structures within the body. These planes are used by medical practitioners to explain the placement of organs, bones, and other structures in relation to one another. Healthcare practitioners may communicate effectively and properly by utilizing exact language and comprehending the planes of the body, resulting in improved patient care.

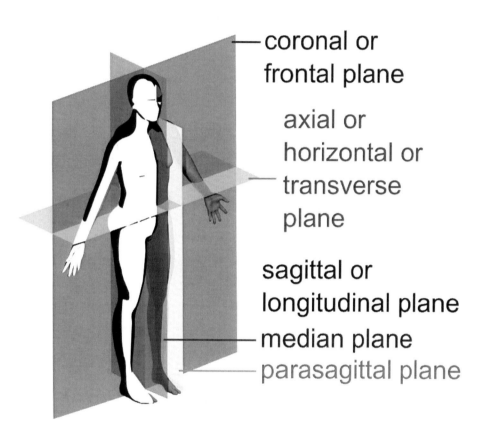

*David Richfield and Mikael Häggström, M.D. and cmglee - Body Planes. The sagittal, frontal (or coronal), and transverse planes are the three most often utilized planes in anatomical and medical imaging – Wikimedia Commons CC BY SA 4.0*

### 2.3.5 Serous Membranes and Body Cavities

The body maintains its internal order by dividing distinct bodily components using diverse structures such as membranes, sheaths, and compartments. The dorsal (posterior) cavity and the ventral (anterior) cavity are the two major compartments of the body. These chambers are critical in safeguarding fragile inside organs and allowing for changes in organ size and form during function. Organs such as the lungs, heart, stomach, and intestines, for example, may expand and contract without causing any disturbance to neighboring tissues or organs.

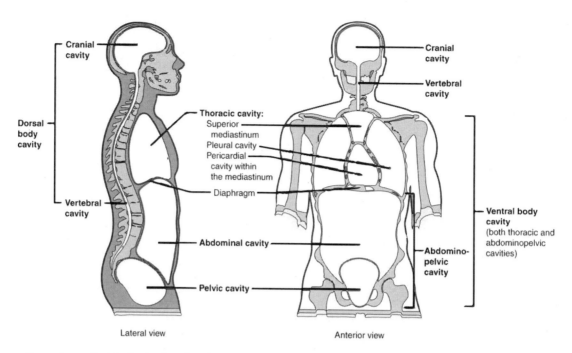

Connexions - *Cavities in the dorsal and ventral body. The thoracic and abdominopelvic cavities, as well as their subdivisions, are included in the ventral cavity. The cranial and spinal cavities are located in the dorsal cavity* Wikimedia Commons CC BY 4.0 and BY 3.0

### 2.3.6 Posterior (Dorsal) and Anterior (Ventral) Cavity Subdivisions

The dorsal and ventral cavities of the body are split into smaller cavities. The brain is housed in the cranial cavity, which is located in the dorsal cavity, whereas the spinal cavity houses the spinal cord. These two chambers are connected in the same way as the brain and spinal cord are connected. The brain and spinal cord are protected by the skull and vertebral column, while cerebrospinal fluid cushions them within the dorsal cavity.

The ventral cavity is divided into two sections: the thoracic cavity and the abdominopelvic cavity. The lungs and heart are housed in the thoracic cavity, which is placed superiorly and is surrounded by the rib cage. The diaphragm divides it from the inferior abdominopelvic cavity, the body's biggest cavity. Although there is no physical membrane that separates the abdominal cavity from the pelvic cavity, it is useful to distinguish between the abdominal cavity, that contains the digestive organs, and the pelvic cavity, which houses the reproductive organs.

### 2.3.7 Quadrants and Abdominal Regions

Health care workers generally divide the cavity into nine areas or four quadrants to improve straightforward communication, such as the location of a patient's stomach discomfort or a suspicious tumor (Look at the figure below).

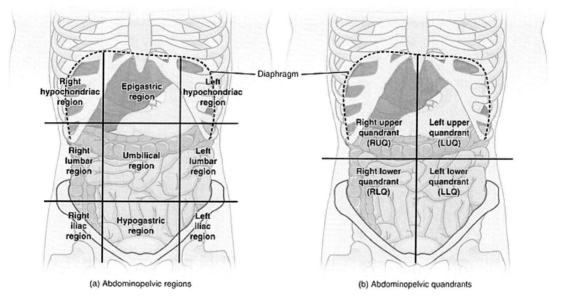

(a) Abdominopelvic regions

(b) Abdominopelvic quadrants

*OpenStax - The Peritoneal Cavity is divided into regions and quadrants. In the peritoneal cavity, there are (a) nine abdominal regions and (b) four abdominal quadrants Wikimedia Commons CC BY 3.0*

To offer a more specific regional approach, draw one horizontal line below the ribs and another above the pelvis, as well as two vertical lines from the middle of each clavicle (collarbone). In contrast, the more typical quadrants technique divides the cavity with one horizontal and one vertical line that connect at the patient's umbilicus (navel).

### 2.3.8 Anterior (Ventral) Body Cavity Membranes

A serosa, referred to as a serous membrane, is a delicate layer that encases the organs and lines the thoracic and abdominopelvic cavities.. The membrane's parietal layer borders the bodily cavity walls (pariet- refers to a cavity wall), whereas the visceral layer covers the organs (the viscera). Between the parietal and visceral layers lies a very thin, fluid-filled serous gap or cavity (Look at the figure below).

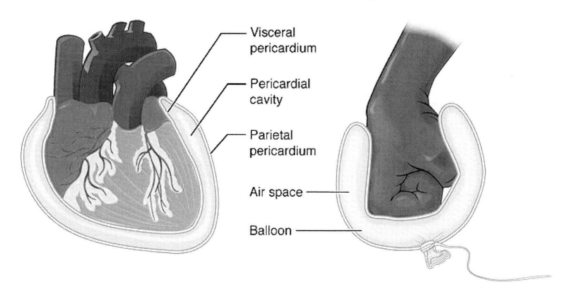

Visceral pericardium

Pericardial cavity

Parietal pericardium

Air space

Balloon

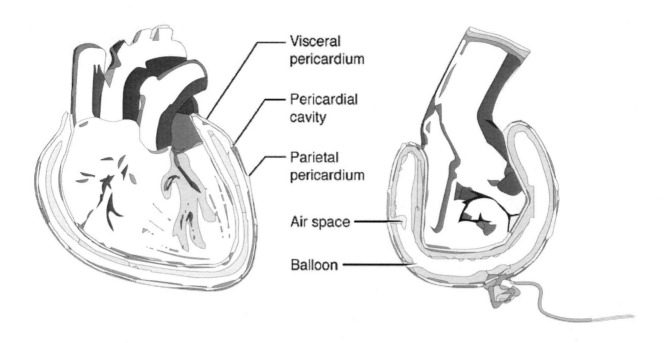

Visceral pericardium

Pericardial cavity

Parietal pericardium

Air space

Balloon

*Connexions - Membrane serous. The pericardial space is lined with serous membrane, which reflects back to cover the heart in the same manner that an underinflated balloon forms two layers around a fist Wikimedia Commons CC BY 3.0*

There are three serous cavities, each with its own membrane. The pleura is the pleural cavity's serous membrane that covers the lungs, the pericardium is the pericardial cavity's serous membrane that surrounds the heart, and the peritoneum is the abdominopelvic cavity's serous membrane that surrounds numerous organs. When internal organs move, such as when the lungs expand or the heart contracts, the serous fluid secreted by the serous membranes minimizes friction between the walls of the cavities and the internal organs. The parietal and visceral serosa both produce the thin, slick serous fluid that minimizes friction as an organ slips past the walls of a hollow.

Pleural fluid minimizes friction between the lungs and the cavity walls in the pleural cavities. Pericardial fluid minimizes friction between the heart and the pericardial sac walls in the pericardial sac. Similar to this, peritoneal fluid lessens friction between the walls of the peritoneal cavity and the abdominal and pelvic organs. The serous membranes shield the viscera they surround by reducing friction that could result in organ inflammation.

# 3 HUMAN SKELETON

## 3.1 INTRODUCTION

The human skeleton, which is made up of many bones and cartilages, is the internal structure of the human body. Bands of fibrous connective tissue called tendons and ligaments attach the bones together. The structure and function of the typical adult human skeleton are the topic of this chapter.

The human skeleton, like that of other vertebrates, may be split into two basic subgroups with separate origins and properties. The spine and most of the skull are included in the first subdivision, the axial. The appendicular division contains the pelvic and pectoral girdles, as well as the bones and cartilages of the limbs. Furthermore, as part of the axial skeleton, this article describes a third subdivision, the visceral, which contains the lower jaw, certain portions of the upper jaw, and the branchial arches, including the hyoid bone.

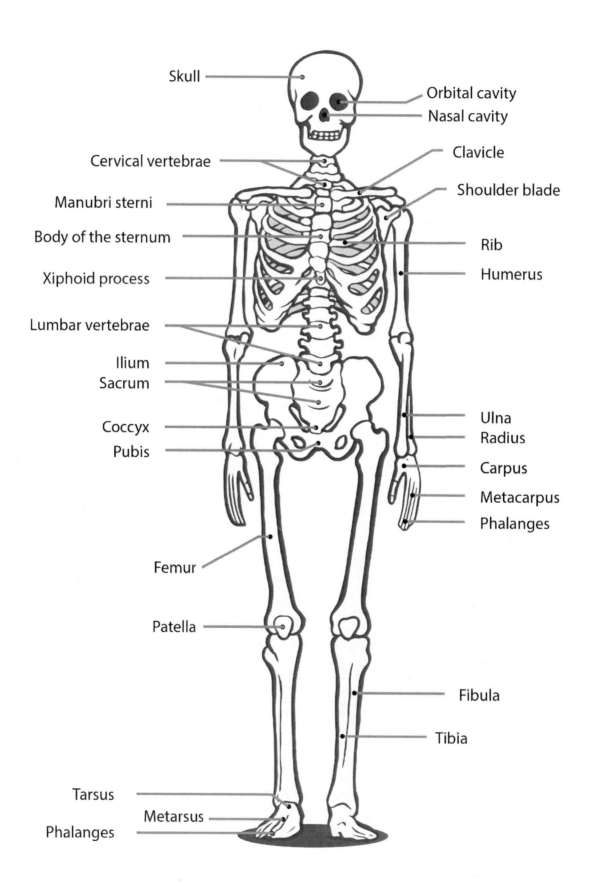

Skull

Orbital cavity

Nasal cavity

Cervical vertebrae

Clavicle

Manubri sterni

Shoulder blade

Body of the sternum

Rib

Humerus

Xiphoid process

Lumbar vertebrae

Ilium

Sacrum

Ulna

Radius

Coccyx

Pubis

Carpus

Metacarpus

Phalanges

Femur

Patella

Fibula

Tibia

Tarsus

Metarsus

Phalanges

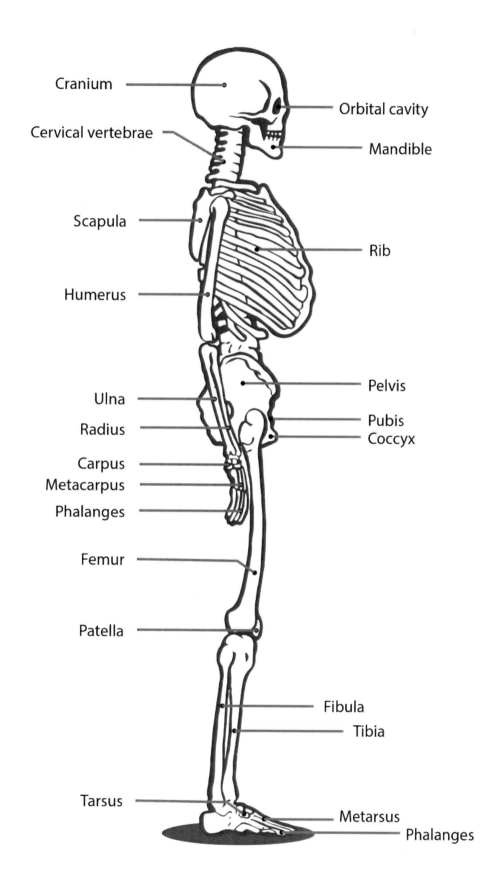

Cranium

Orbital cavity

Cervical vertebrae

Mandible

Scapula

Rib

Humerus

Pelvis

Ulna

Radius

Pubis

Coccyx

Carpus

Metacarpus

Phalanges

Femur

Patella

Fibula

Tibia

Tarsus

Metarsus

Phalanges

When the subdivisions of the skeleton are compared to the soft tissues of the body, such as the neurological, digestive, respiratory, circulatory, and muscular systems, it is clear that the skeleton's functions fall into three categories: support, protection, and mobility. The most rudimentary and oldest function is support, and the axial skeleton was the first to develop to serve this purpose. The fundamental support for the trunk is the vertebral column, which corresponds to the notochord in lower creatures.

The central nervous system is predominantly housed inside the axial skeleton, with the skull protecting the brain and the spinal cord being protected by the vertebral column, neural arches, and bone intervening ligaments.

The upright posture is one of the characteristics that separates humans from other mammals. The human body is like a walking tower, moving on pillars represented by the legs. This position has provided tremendous benefits, including releasing the arms for a variety of purposes. However, the upright position has caused a variety of mechanical issues, notably with weight-bearing, necessitating skeletal system adjustments.

Protecting the heart, lungs, and other chest organs is a distinct challenge than protecting the central nervous system. To accommodate motion, expansion, and contraction, these organs require a flexible and elastic protective covering. This covering is provided by the bony thoracic basket, also known as the rib cage, which functions as the skeleton of the chest wall or thorax. The ribs' attachment to the sternum is secondary, made possible by relatively elastic rib cartilages. During breathing and other activities, small joints between the ribs and vertebrae allow the ribs to glide on the vertebrae, with mobility restricted by ligamentous attachments between the ribs and vertebrae.

When the subdivisions of the skeleton are compared to the soft tissues of the body, such as the neurological, digestive, respiratory, circulatory, and muscular systems, it is clear that the skeleton's functions fall into three categories: support, protection, and mobility. The most rudimentary and oldest function is support, and the axial skeleton was the first to develop to serve this purpose. The fundamental support for the trunk is the vertebral column, which corresponds to the notochord in lower creatures.

The central nervous system is predominantly housed inside the axial skeleton, with the skull protecting the brain and the spinal cord being protected by the vertebral column, neural arches, and bone intervening ligaments.

The upright posture is one of the characteristics that separates humans from other mammals. The human body is like a walking tower, moving on pillars represented by the legs. This position has provided tremendous benefits, including releasing the arms for a variety of purposes. However, the upright position has caused a variety of mechanical issues, notably with weight-bearing, necessitating skeletal system adjustments.

Protecting the heart, lungs, and other chest organs is a distinct challenge than protecting the central nervous system. These organs need an elastic and flexible covering to allow for motion, expansion, and contraction. The bony thoracic basket, sometimes referred to as the rib cage, serves as the skeleton of the chest wall, or thorax, and provides this covering. The ribs' attachment to the sternum is secondary, made possible by relatively elastic rib cartilages. During breathing and other activities, small joints between the ribs and vertebrae allow the ribs to glide on the vertebrae, with mobility restricted by ligamentous attachments between the ribs and vertebrae.

## 3.2   SKELETAL AXES AND VISCERA

### 3.2.1   The cranium

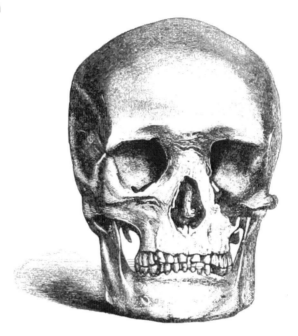

*Human Skeleton*

The cranium, which houses the brain, is sometimes known as the braincase. This word, however, can be deceptive because the cranium is also linked to the sense organs of sight, hearing, smell, and taste, as well as other structures.

The skull is made up of two types of bones that developed in separate ways: cartilaginous or substitution bones, which replace cartilage in the overall shape of the bone, and membrane bones, which form inside layers of connective tissue. Substitution bones constitute the cranium's floor, while membrane bones form the sides and roof.

Because of changes in bone thickness and the amount of air pockets or sinuses, the capacity of the cranial cavity varies greatly but is not directly equal to the size of the skull. While the floor of the cranial cavity is rough and uneven, the landmarks and structural features are typically constant throughout skulls.

The cranium is the upper section of the skull, with the facial bones located beneath it. It is made up of several big bones, such as the frontal, sphenoid, two temporal bones, two parietal bones, and the occipital bone. The frontal bone sits behind the forehead and links to minor bones in the nasal bridge, the zygomatic bone, the sphenoid bone, and the maxillary bones. The frontal bone's horizontal component extends back between the nasal and zygomatic bones to create a piece of the orbit's roof, protecting the eye and its associated structures.

Each parietal bone has a four-sided shape and contributes significantly to the cranium's side walls. They communicate with the frontal, sphenoid, temporal, and occipital bones, as well as their opposite-side equivalents. These bones are largely cranial, having less relationship to other structures than the other cranial bones.

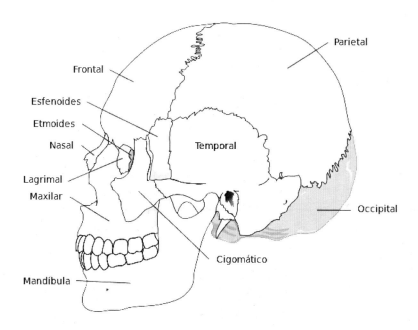

*LadyofHats - Anatomy of the Adult Skull - Bones and Sutures Wikimedia Commons.*

## Interior of the cranium

The inside of the skull is richly detailed, reflecting the forms of the softer tissues in touch with the bones.

The vault's inside surface is quite basic. The superior longitudinal venous sinus, a big route for venous blood, is located in the midline front-to-back groove along the sagittal suture. Pacchionian bodies, which allow the venous system to absorb cerebrospinal fluid, are indicated by depressions on each side of the groove. The skull protects the thin-walled venous sinuses, which are all located within the cranial cavity. They are, however, so close to the bones in many locations that a fracture or penetrating cut can rupture the sinus wall, causing blood that often becomes trapped under the outer and hardest brain covering, the dura mater, resulting in a subdural hematoma.

The middle meningeal artery and its branches that give blood to the brain coverings generate markings on the interior surface of the sphenoid projection, known as the larger wing, as well as on the parietal and temporal bones. Extradural hematoma, a mass of blood between the dura mater and the bone, can result from damage to these veins.

The base of the skull has a complicated appearance, with three prominent depressions, or fossae, arranged in a descending stair-step pattern from front to back. The fossae are connected to key regions of the brain and are rigidly segregated by the margins of the cranial bones. The frontal lobes of the cerebrum (the vast forward region of the brain) sleep in the anterior cranial fossa. The temporal lobes of the cerebrum are housed in the middle cranial fossa, which is separated into two lateral parts by a central bone prominence. The posterior cranial fossa houses the cerebellum (a mass of brain tissue behind the brain stem and underneath the cerebrum's back section) as well as the front and middle portions of the brain stem. Major regions of the brain are partly encased by the cranial wall bones.

The pituitary gland is located in the middle cerebral fossa's central eminence, which has a saddle-like seat known as the sella turcica. The dorsum sellae, or rear section of this seat, is wall-like. The pituitary gland is hidden under the brain coverings and is only accessible to the outside of the cranium via blood vessels.

The cerebrum's temporal lobes are positioned in the deep lateral parts of the middle cranial fossa. The fossa also has various openings, including the superior orbital fissure and the foramen rotundum, which allow the maxillary nerve to pass through. The mandibular nerve connects to the lower jaw through the foramen ovale, whereas the middle meningeal artery provides blood to the dura mater through the foramen spinosum.

The posterior cranial fossa is situated above the spinal column and the rear of the neck muscles. The foramen magnum, the aperture through which the brain and spinal cord join, is located at the bottom of this fossa. The clivus is a large, smooth bony surface located between the foramen magnum's front edge and the base of the dorsum sellae. The brain stem's bridgelike pons and pyramid-like medulla oblongata reside on the clivus, isolated from the bone only by their coverings. Near the foramen magnum, there are ridges for the attachment of dura mater folds.

The sidewalls of the posterior cranial fossa have two transverse grooves that are partly isolated from the mastoid air cells behind the ear by exceedingly thin bone. The jugular foramina are apertures that allow vast blood channels known as the sigmoid sinuses, as well as the 9th (glossopharyngeal), 10th (vagus), and 11th (spinal accessory) cranial nerves, to exit the cranial cavity, to pass through.

The arteries and cranial nerves are vulnerable to damage at the cranial cavity's entrances and in certain places, such as around the mastoid air cells. Mastoiditis, an infection of the mastoid air cells, can cause enough bone disintegration to allow disease-bearing organisms to enter the cranial cavity and cause catastrophic consequences.

### 3.2.2   The hyoid: an illustration of the anchoring function

The hyoid bone's primary purpose is to act as a tongue anchor. This bone is placed in the front of the neck, between the lower jaw and the biggest cartilage of the larynx, near the base of the tongue. The hyoid bone, unlike other bones in the body, does not articulate with other bones and simply functions as an anchor.

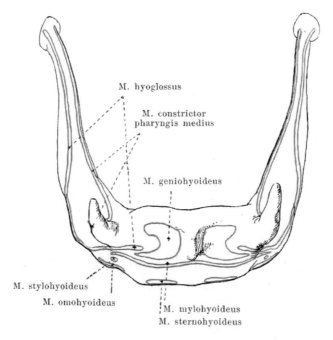

*Werner Spalteholz - Human hyoid bone Wikimedia Commons*

The hyoid bone is U-shaped and consists of a body and four horns. The bigger cornua has the larger horns, whereas the lesser cornua has the smaller horns. The middle section or base of the U-shape is formed by the bone's body.

The hyoid bone, tongue, and larynx all move rapidly upward during swallowing. This movement is required for the swallowing process to work correctly. The hyoid bone is particularly important in speech and singing because it controls the position and movement of the tongue. Any abnormalities or injuries to the hyoid bone might impair the function of the tongue and larynx, resulting in swallowing and speech issues.

The limbs of the U-shaped hyoid bone form the larger cornua. The big sternocleidomastoid muscles in the neck often overlap their outer ends. The smaller cornua are tiny projections that form at the body and greater cornua connections.

The hyoid bone, to which some tongue muscles are linked, is important in tongue movement. The hyoglossus muscles, for example, arise from the whole length of the larger cornua and the hyoid body. They are implanted into the tongue's posterior half or more of its sides. When these muscles contract, they depress the tongue and expand the oral cavity, with the hyoid bone acting as an anchor.

The geniohyoid muscles arise near the junction of the two parts of the lower jaw. The fibers of the muscles extend downward and backward, near to the central line, to be inserted into the hyoid bone's body. The hyoid bone is pulled upward and forward by the contraction of these muscles.

The sternohyoid muscles are lengthy muscles that go up and toward each other in the neck from the breastbone and collarbone. They fit into the centre of the hyoid bone's bottom border. During swallowing, these muscles depress the hyoid bone and larynx.

The hyoid bone is connected to several muscles, including the mylohyoid muscles, which form a diaphragm-like structure for the floor of the mouth, the thyrohyoid muscle, which arises from the larynx's largest cartilage, and the omohyoid muscle, which arises from the upper margin of the shoulder blade and the suprascapular ligament.

The hyoid bone and its muscle attachments have been described to a ship moored "fore and aft," and they play an important role in mastication, swallowing, and voice production.

The geniohyoid and mylohyoid muscles concurrently raise the bone and the floor of the mouth while swallowing, with aid from the stylohyoid and digastric muscles. The tongue pushes on the palate, pushing food backward.

### 3.2.3   The various functions of the facial bones

#### 3.2.3.1   The upper jaws
The maxillae, often known as the upper jaws, are the largest portion of the face skeleton. However, their duties and scope extend beyond just supplementing the lower jaw. They also form the middle and bottom parts of the eye socket and house the nose aperture between them, which is placed below the tiny nasal bones. They also produce the anterior nasal spine, a sharp protrusion in the middle of the nasal aperture's bottom edge.

The infraorbital foramen is a hole on the floor of the eye socket that houses the infraorbital branch of the maxillary nerve, the second division of the fifth cranial nerve. This foramen lies immediately below the bottom edge of the eye socket.

The lower section of each maxilla is formed by the alveolar border, which contains the sockets or alveoli in which the upper teeth reside. Furthermore, each maxilla has a lateral projection known as the zygomatic process, which connects to the zygomatic or malar bone (cheekbone).

### 3.2.3.2  The lower jaw

The lower jaw, or mandible, begins as two distinct bones on the left and right sides of the head. However, during the second year of life, they fuse together at the midline to create a single bone. The mandible's body is the horizontal center piece on either side, with the top portion creating the alveolar edge, which corresponds to the maxillae. The chin is a distinguishing feature of the human skull that protrudes from the bottom half of the body near the midline. The mental foramen is an aperture on each side of the chin for the mental branch of the mandibular nerve, the third division of the fifth cranial nerve.

The ascending sections of the mandible are called rami (branches). The joints that allow the lower jaw to move are placed between the rounded knob, or condyle, at the upper rear corner of each ramus and a depression in each temporal bone known as the glenoid fossa. The coronoid process, which is a sharp protrusion at the top of each ramus and in front, is not a joint. However, it is connected to the temporalis muscle, which helps to seal the jaws. Each ramus has a wide, obliquely situated aperture into the mandibular canal, which is a route for nerves, arteries, and veins.

The zygomatic arch, which creates the cheekbone, is made up of three bones: the maxilla in front, the zygomatic bone in the center, and a temporal bone projection in the back. The strong masseter muscle has its bone origin in the zygomatic arch. The masseter muscle descends from the zygomatic arch to enter on the outer side of the mandible, sharing the role of raising the jaw with other muscles such as the temporalis muscle and the lateral and medial pterygoid muscles for biting.

## 3.3   The Spine

The evolution of the human species has demanded the adaptation and modification of the human skeletal system, resulting in the particular structure of the vertebral column. This suggests that the human spinal column has evolved to accommodate the necessity for upright posture.

### 3.3.1   The vertebral column

The vertebral column, though frequently referred to as a column, is actually a spiral spring shaped like the letter S. The spinal column of a kid is generally straight at birth, but curvatures emerge when the supporting roles of the vertebral column in humans, such as holding up the trunk, keeping the head erect, and anchoring the limbs, are established.

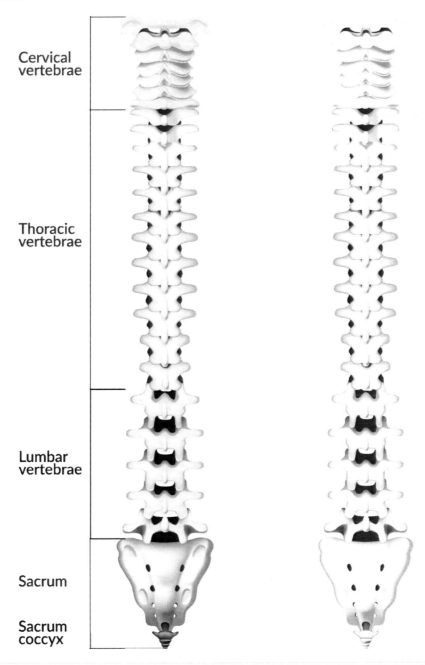

Cervical vertebrae

Thoracic vertebrae

Lumbar vertebrae

Sacrum

Sacrum coccyx

The spinal column's S-shaped curve absorbs the shocks of walking on hard surfaces, whereas a straight column would carry jarring shocks directly from the pelvic girdle to the brain. Furthermore, the curvature tackles the issue of bearing the viscera's weight. The viscera would pull the column forward in an upright animal with a straight column. Concavities in the thoracic and pelvic areas provide for more room for the viscera.

The S-curvature of the spinal column also influences weight distribution throughout the body. The top sector supports the head, the center sector the thoracic viscera, and the lower sector the abdominal viscera. The weight burden would be highest at the base and rise from the head downward if the column were straight. Furthermore, the S-curvature protects the vertebral column from fracture since the doubly bent spring arrangement is less prone to fracture than a straight column.

The skeleton's protective role is most visible in connection to the central nervous system, while it is also necessary for the heart, lungs, and several other organs. Because of the restricted amount of mobility and expansion required by its component parts, as well as specific physiological adaptations related to circulation, cerebrospinal fluid, and the meninges - the coverings of the brain and spinal cord - the central nervous system is well protected. The pituitary gland, or hypophysis, is further protected by the cranium's protective enclosure of the brain.

### 3.3.2 The spinal cord

The spinal cord, which carries nerve fibers that flow to and from the brain, is positioned similarly to a candle in a lantern in respect to the spinal column. The meninges, cerebrospinal fluid, and some fat and connective tissue normally occupy a large amount of space between the neurological and skeletal structures. The front is occupied by the vertebral bodies and intervertebral disks, while the neural arches of each vertebra surround and protect the cord from the back and sides. Interlaminar ligaments, also known as ligamenta flava, are elastic connective tissue sheets that run between the neural arches. The forward bending of portion of the column produces separation between the laminae and spines of the neural arches of contiguous vertebrae, sacrificing some protective function to allow for mobility. The lumbar puncture (spinal tap) needle enters the subarachnoid space via the ligamenta flava of the lower lumbar region (the small of the back).

In addition to its support and protective duties, the vertebral column is important in muscle anchoring. Many of the muscles related to it are structured in such a manner that they may move the column or different portions of it, some of which are superficial and others deep-lying. The erector spinae, a big and important muscle, keeps the spine upright. It starts in the sacrum, a big triangular bone at the base of the spinal column, and travels up to create a muscular mass on either side of the lumbar vertebrae's spines. It then splits into three columns that climb over the back of the chest. While narrow strips of the muscle are inserted into the vertebrae and ribs, it does not stop there; new slips emerge from these same bones and continue up into the neck until one of the divisions, the longissimus capitis, ultimately reaches the skull.

Small muscles travel between the transverse processes of neighboring vertebrae, between the vertebral spines, and from the transverse process to the spine, allowing the segmented bony column to move freely.

The spinal column's anchoring role is critical for the muscles that originate from the trunk, either wholly or partially from the column or from ligaments linked to it, and insert on the bones of the arms and legs. The latissimus dorsi (which drags the arm backward and downward while turning it inward), trapezius (which rotates the shoulder blade), rhomboideus, and levator scapulae (which lifts and lowers the shoulder blade) are the most crucial for the arms. The psoas muscles (placed in the loin) are the most crucial for the legs.

## 3.4   THE RIB CAGE

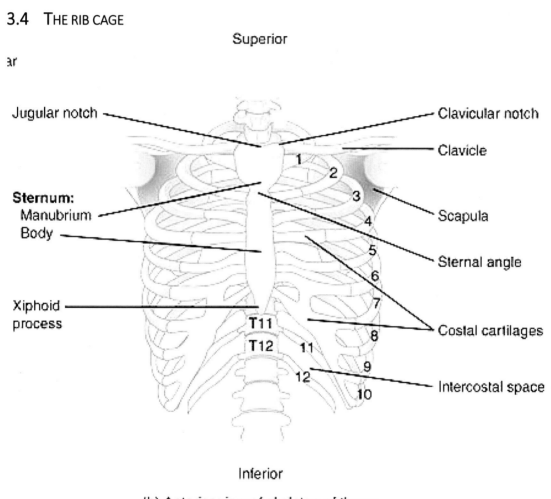

(b) Anterior view of skeleton of thorax

*OpenStax College Wikimedia Commons*

The thoracic basket, commonly known as the rib cage, is made up of the 12 thoracic vertebrae, 24 ribs, and the sternum or breastbone. The ribs are bent and compressed bone bars, with each consecutive rib becoming more open in curvature as it progresses from the first or topmost rib. A rib's angle, or point of greatest change in curvature, is positioned several inches from the rib's head, which forms a connection with the vertebrae.

True ribs are the first seven ribs that are linked to the breastbone by costal cartilages. The costal cartilages of the other five ribs, known as false ribs, are joined to the cartilage above them. The last two ribs are known as floating ribs because their cartilages finish in the abdominal wall muscle rather than being linked to

the sternum.

The rib cage protects the thoracic organs, including the heart and lungs, and aids in breathing by extending and contracting to transfer air into and out of the lungs. The rib cage may expand and contract due to the curvature of the ribs and the flexibility of the costal cartilages.

The rib cage is semirigid yet expansile, expanding in size due to the activity of many muscles. When the rib cage expands, the pressure inside the lungs falls below the pressure outside the lungs, prompting air to rush into the lungs to restore balance. This is known as inspiration or breathing in. Expiration, on the other hand, is caused by the relaxation of the respiratory muscles and the elastic recoil of the lungs, fibrous ligaments, and tendons linked to the thoracic skeleton.

The diaphragm, which divides the chest and belly and has a wide origin from the rib cage and spinal column, is one of the primary breathing muscles. The arrangement of the bottom five ribs allows for the expansion of the lower rib cage and the movement of the diaphragm, both of which are required for breathing.

The respiratory center in the brainstem controls the breathing process, adjusting the pace and depth of breathing to fulfill the body's oxygen requirement. Breathing is an essential mechanism that ensures the body's cells get the oxygen they need to function properly.

## 3.5 The Appendicular Skeleton

### 3.5.1 Pectoral girdle and pelvic girdle

Humans have homologous upper and lower extremities that have a shared origin and are patterned on the same fundamental layout. These extremes provide various opportunities for comparison and contrast. Nonetheless, the two pairs of limbs differ significantly due to their extensive evolutionary history and major variations in function.

Girdles are the sections of the extremities closest to the body's axis and serve to link the free extremity (arm or leg) to the axis, either directly via the skeleton or indirectly through muscle attachments. The sacroiliac joint connects the pelvic girdle to the spinal column. On the continuous surfaces of the ilium (rear and top section of the hip bone) and sacrum (part of the vertebral column immediately associated with the hip bone), thin plates of cartilage occur. These bones are tightly packed together, with irregular masses of softer fibrocartilage connecting the articular cartilages. Fibrous attachments occur between the bones in the top and lower regions of the joint, and the joint cavity contains a modest quantity of synovial fluid. Strong ligaments connect the pelvic girdle to the vertebral column, including the anterior and posterior sacroiliac and interosseous ligaments. These fibrous attachments are the major limiting factors of joint mobility, although muscle tone in this area is also important in avoiding or resolving frequent sacroiliac problems.

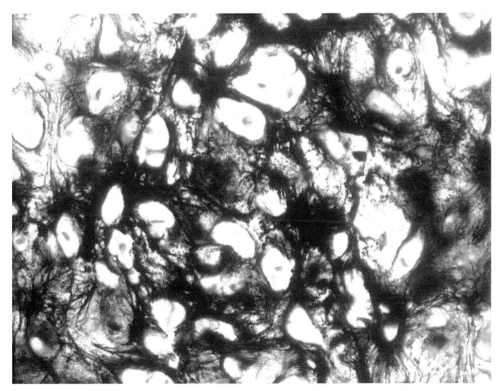

*Cartilage*

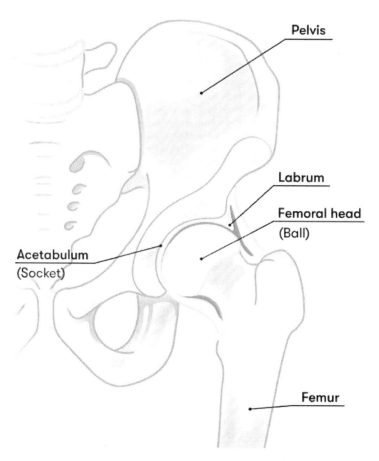

Pelvis

Labrum

Femoral head
(Ball)

Acetabulum
(Socket)

Femur

The pelvic girdle is initially made up of three bones that merge throughout early adulthood and contribute to the acetabulum. The acetabulum is a deep cavity that houses the femoral head, or thighbone. The ilium is the flared top half of the girdle, whereas the pubis is the lower anterior component that connects to the ilium at the midline. The ischium is the girdle's lowest posterior section. Each ischial bone has a tuberosity, or protrusion, and the body rests on these tuberosities while seated.

The pectoral girdle, or upper extremity girdle, is made up of the scapula (shoulder blade) and the clavicle (collarbone). The glenoid cavity, a depression in the scapula, houses the head of the humerus, the long bone of the upper arm. The pectoral girdle, unlike the pelvic girdle, is not attached to the spinal column by ligamentous attachments and has no connection with any component of the body axis. The trapezius, rhomboids, and levator scapulae are the only muscles that link the scapula to the rib cage, whereas the serratus anterior connects the scapula to the rib cage. The pectoral girdle, particularly the scapula, has a far larger range of motion than the pelvic girdle.

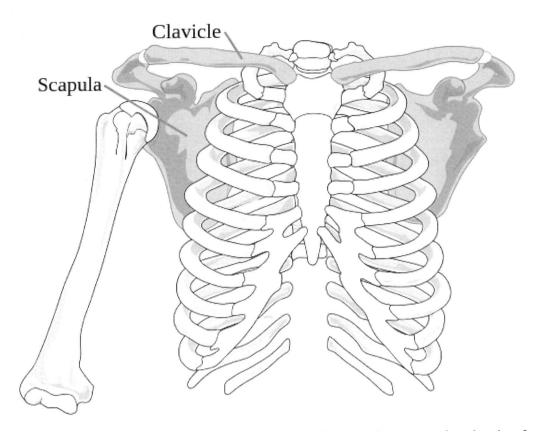

Clavicle

Scapula

In terms of the shallowness of the glenoid fossa relative to the depth of the acetabulum, the function of the pectoral girdle differs from that of the pelvic girdle. Although the glenoid labrum, a fibrocartilage lip, deepens the receptacle for the head of the humerus to some extent, the free upper extremity has a far larger range of motion than the lower extremity. This increased range of motion comes at a larger risk of dislocation, making the shoulder the most often dislocated joint in the body.

### 3.5.2 Arm and leg long bones

In the arms and legs, the humerus and femur are comparable bones. Although their pieces are similar in general, their architectures have evolved to serve various purposes. The humeral head is approximately hemispherical, while the femoral head is roughly two-thirds of a sphere. In addition, a strong ligament connects the femoral head to the acetabulum, strengthening and securing its place.

In comparison to the femoral neck, the anatomical neck of the humerus has a small constriction. The femoral neck is a considerably more defined section that extends from the head and joins the shaft at a 125° angle. In reality, the femoral neck is considered a member of the shaft both developmentally and functionally. The entire body's weight is directed through the femoral heads, down their necks, and into the shaft. The bone structure within the head, neck, and upper section of the shaft of the femur is noteworthy, demonstrating the weight-bearing issues involved in maintaining an upright position. An engineer who has dealt with similar issues would surely be amazed.

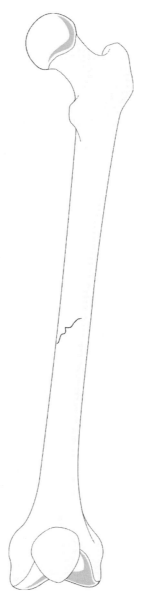

Each forearm and lower leg has two long bones. The forearm contains the radius and the ulna, which are found on the thumb side of the forearm. The tibia (shinbone) and fibula are located in the lower leg. The tibia is represented by the radius, and the fibula by the ulna. The knee joint is not only the biggest but also the most complicated joint in the body. The femur and tibia are the only bones engaged in this joint, albeit the smaller fibula bone is carried along in the joint's flexion, extension, and mild rotation. During fetal development, the relatively thin fibula is significantly thicker relative to the tibia than it is in the adult skeleton.

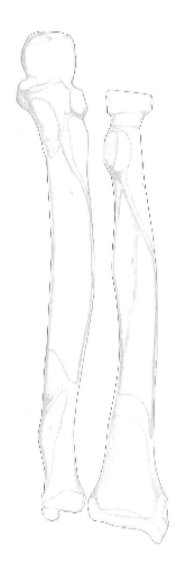

The humerus and ulna form a genuine hinge joint at the elbow, enabling only flexion and extension motions. The olecranon, a prominent ulnar projection, fits into the well-defined olecranon fossa, a humeral depression.

The radius is shorter than the ulna and has a unique disk-shaped head that articulates with the humerus's head (capitulum). A strong annular ligament binds the radius head against the notch on the ulna's side. Despite being linked to the ulna, the head of the radius has the ability to spin, enabling the shaft and outer end of the radius to swing in an arc. The radius and ulna are parallel in the supination position, the palm facing forward, and the thumb is distant from the body. The radius and ulna are crossed in the pronation position, the palm is facing back, and the thumb is adjacent to the body. There are no leg movements similar to supination and pronation of the arm.

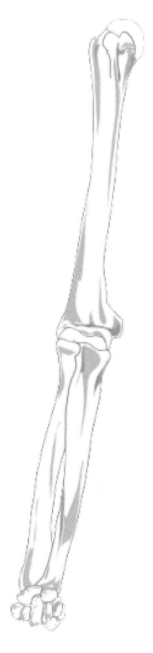

### 3.5.3 The hands and feet

The carpus, or wrist, is made up of eight tiny carpal bones grouped in two rows of four each. Because of the angle of the foot to the leg and its weight-bearing function, the ankle, or tarsus, contains seven bones organized in a more intricate manner. The calcaneus is the heel bone, pointing downward and backward, whereas the talus is the tarsus keystone, with the superior surface articulating with the heel bone.

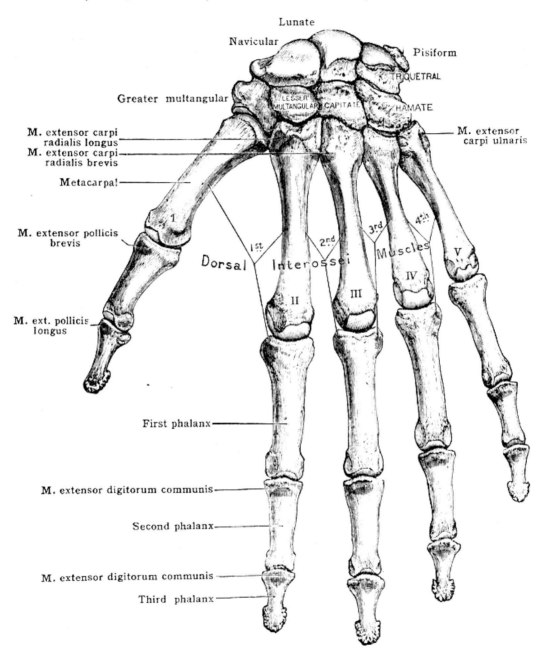

*Morris' human anatomy (1933)*
*Wikimedia Commons*

The outside component of the skeleton of the arms and legs is specialized and consists of extended regions made up of chains, or linear series, of tiny bones. These outer sections have had a complicated evolutionary history, initially passing through a period in which all four would have acted as weight-bearing extremities, as in quadrupeds in general. Then, like in lesser primates or "four-handed folk," all four were suited for arboreal existence. Finally, the adoption of an upright posture relegated the distal sections of the rear, now lower, extremities to the job of feet, while the front, now upper, extremities developed exceptional manipulating abilities and are known as hands. It is difficult to say when a foot becomes a hand in the primate lineage, and one could argue that raccoons, squirrels, and other nonprimates have hands as well.

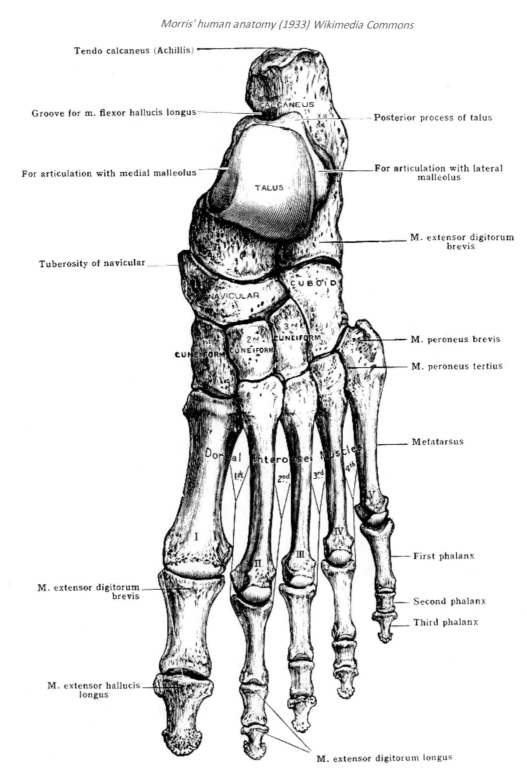

*Morris' human anatomy (1933) Wikimedia Commons*

The metatarsal bones of the foot are actually bigger than the metacarpal bones of the hand. The tarsals and metatarsals work together to produce the foot's arches, which give it strength and allow it to operate as a lever. The form of each bone and its connection to the others are tailored to this function.

The bases of the phalanges, or toe bones, are larger than those of the equivalent bones in the hand, but the shafts are considerably thinner. The foot's middle and outer phalanges are shorter than the fingers'. The phalanges of the big toe have unique characteristics.

The thumb and its structure, which includes the first metacarpal bone and two phalanges, make the hand a unique instrument for delicate and diverse movements. Flexion, extension, abduction (the capacity to pull away from the first finger), and adduction (the ability to move forward of the fingers) are all free motions of the thumb, which are likewise exerted to varied degrees by the big toe. The thumb, on the other hand, has a unique movement known as opposition, which allows it to be brought across, or opposed to, the palm and the tips of the slightly flexed fingers. This action is the foundation for manipulating tools, weapons, and instruments, as well as the delicate and precise motions necessary for tasks like writing, sketching, and playing musical instruments. The capacity to resist the thumb in this manner is one of the trademarks of the human hand and is critical to our ability to manage our surroundings and construct complicated tools and technology.

# 4 THE MUSCULAR SYSTEM

The human muscular system is made up of muscles that are under voluntary control and help in movement, posture, and balance of the skeletal system. Muscles in vertebrates, including humans, are divided into three types: striated muscle (or skeletal muscle), smooth muscle, and cardiac muscle. Smooth muscle is present in the walls of blood arteries as well as organs such as the urine bladder, intestines, and stomach. Cardiac muscle, which makes up the majority of the heart, is in charge of rhythmic contractions and is also under involuntary control. With few variations, the organization of smooth and cardiac muscle in humans is similar to that of other animals. This classification enables a clear knowledge of the many roles and properties of the different types of muscles in the human body.

The parts that follow offer a fundamental framework for comprehending the primary muscle groups and their functions as well as the overall human muscular structure. These muscle groups operate together in unison to control the human body's motions.

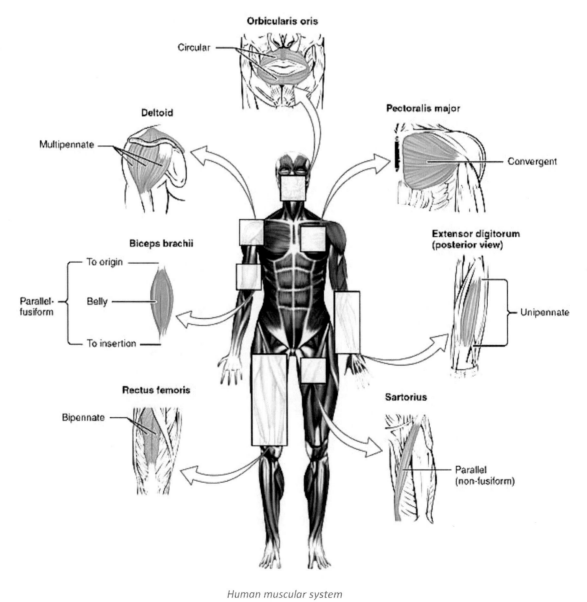

*Human muscular system*

## 4.1   THE NECK

Rotation, flexion, extension, and side bending (also known as lateral flexion, which includes moving the ear towards the shoulder) are the movements of the neck. The direction of movement can be either ipsilateral (moving towards the side of the contracting muscle) or contralateral (moving away from the side of the contracting muscle).

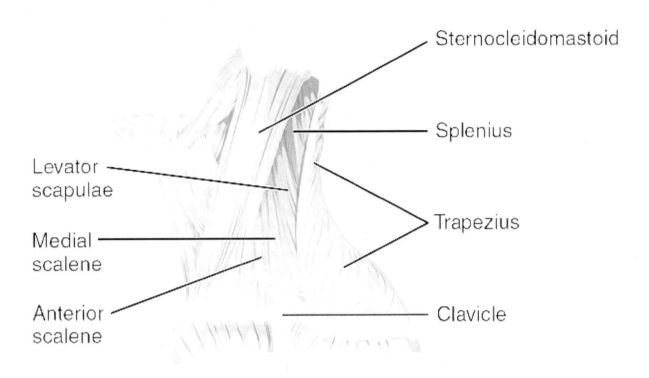

*OpenStax College - Neck Muscles Wikimedia Commons CC BY 3.0*

The sternocleidomastoid muscle is the primary performer of rotation in the cervical spine. This muscle turns the neck to the other side and bends it to the same side. Furthermore, both sternocleidomastoid muscles collaborate to bend the neck and raise the sternum during forceful inhalation. The anterior and middle scalene muscles also help in rotation and elevating the first rib. The splenius capitis and splenius cervicis, situated near the back of the neck, are in charge of head rotation.

Another important movement of the cervical spine is side bending, which involves the sternocleidomastoid muscle. The posterior scalene muscles, located on the neck's bottom sides, bend the neck to the same side and raise the second rib. Splenix capitis and splenius cervicis are also involved in neck side bending. The erector spinae muscles, which include the iliocostalis, longissimus, and spinalis, run the length of the back. The three muscles work together to bend the neck to the same side.

The motion of moving the chin towards the chest is referred to as neck flexion, and it is predominantly achieved by the sternocleidomastoid muscles. The front of the neck muscles longus colli and longus capitis also help in neck flexion. Neck extension, on the other hand, entails extending the head rearward and is carried out by many of the same muscles as other neck motions. The splenius cervicis, splenius capitis, iliocostalis, longissimus, and spinalis muscles are among them.

## 4.2 THE BACK

Many muscles in the back play an important part in the mobility of the neck and shoulders. Furthermore, the spinal cord, which innervates almost all muscles in the body, is protected by the axial skeleton, which runs vertically through the back.

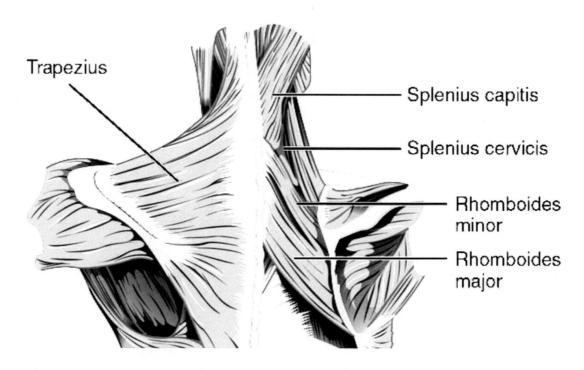

*OpenStax College - Neck Back Muscles Wikimedia Commons CC BY 3.0*

Several muscles in the back are responsible for distinct back motions. The erector spinae muscles, for example, extend (bend rearward) and side bend the back. The back is additionally extended by the semispinalis dorsi and semispinalis capitis muscles. Small vertebral muscles, such as the multifidi and rotators, assist in rotating, extending, and side bending the back.

Through its stabilizing function at the insertion site on the 12th rib (the last of the floating ribs), the quadratus lumborum muscle in the lower back side bends the lumbar spine and aids in air intake. The scapula (shoulder blade) is elevated by the trapezius muscle, which runs from the back of the neck to the center of the back, the rhomboid major and minor muscles in the upper back, and the levator scapulae muscle, which runs down the side and back of the neck.

## 4.3 THE SHOULDER

The shoulder is a complicated ball-and-socket joint composed of the humeral head, the clavicle (collarbone), and the scapula. It may move in a variety of directions, including flexion, extension, abduction, adduction, internal rotation, and exterior rotation.

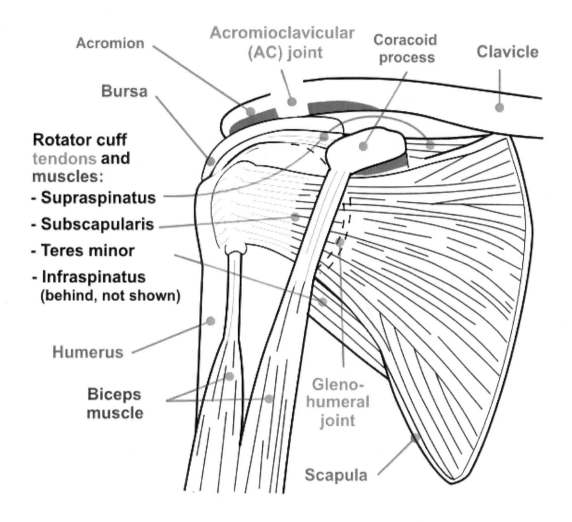

*National Institute Of Arthritis And Musculoskeletal And Skin Diseases - Shoulder Muscles Wikimedia Commons*

Shoulder flexion is the forward movement of the shoulder, as when reaching for an object. The deltoid muscle at the top of the arm, the pectoralis major muscle in the chest, the coracobrachialis muscle on the inside of the upper arm, and the biceps brachii muscles on the front of the upper arm all work together to make this movement possible.

Shoulder extension is the inverse of flexion, and it involves moving the arm squarely behind the body, as when receiving a baton in a relay race. The activities of many muscles, including the deltoid muscle, the latissimus dorsi muscle in the back, the teres major muscle in the armpit area, and the triceps muscle at the rear of the upper arm, are principally responsible for this movement. The triceps muscle is made up of three heads that originate from various surfaces but share the same insertion at the ulnar olecranon process, and they work together to extend the elbow.

Shoulder adduction and abduction are responsible for bringing the arm closer to and away from the body, respectively. Imagine someone performing jumping jacks to visualize these motions. The pectoralis major, latissimus dorsi, teres major, triceps, and coracobrachialis muscles are principally responsible for adduction. The two primary abductors of the shoulder are the deltoid and supraspinatus muscles, which run along the scapula in the back.

The deltoid, teres minor, and infraspinatus muscles are principally responsible for external rotation of the shoulder, as shown in a tennis backhand stroke. Internal rotation, on the other hand, happens while reaching into a rear pocket and is the inverse of external rotation. Several muscles, including the pectoralis major, latissimus dorsi, deltoid, teres major, and subscapularis, work together to produce this movement. The subscapularis muscle is located on the scapula's anterior surface.

The rotator cuff is made up of the teres minor, subscapularis, supraspinatus, and infraspinatus muscles, and it is responsible for stabilizing the humeral head in the ball-and-socket shoulder joint. These muscles are frequently damaged in adults, especially those who execute repetitive overhead activities like tossing a baseball or painting a ceiling. Some rotator cuff tendons travel beneath the acromion, a bony protrusion at the distal end of the scapula. The tendons and subacromial bursae (fluid-filled sacs beneath the acromion) are sensitive to compression and squeezing in this posture, resulting to shoulder impingement syndrome.

## 4.4 THE ARM

In addition to assisting with shoulder mobility, the upper arm muscles also help with forearm motions. Forearm flexion, or moving the hand closer to the shoulder by decreasing the angle between the forearm and the upper arm, is primarily accomplished by the biceps brachii, brachialis (located beneath the biceps brachii in the upper arm), and brachioradialis (originating from the humerus). The coracobrachialis and flexor muscles located in the anterior compartment of the forearm (also known as the flexor compartment), such as the pronator teres, flexor carpi radialis, flexor digitorum superficialis, palmaris longus, and flexor carpi ulnaris, also contribute to forearm flexion.

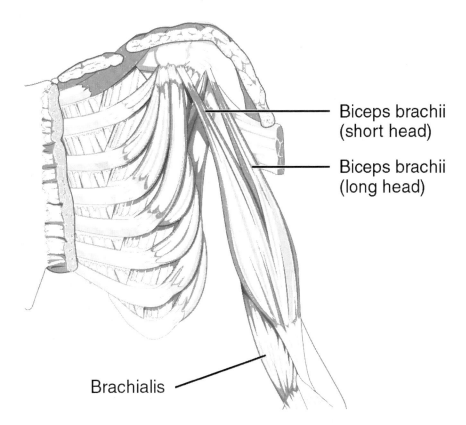

Biceps brachii (short head)

Biceps brachii (long head)

Brachialis

Left upper arm muscles (anterior lateral view)

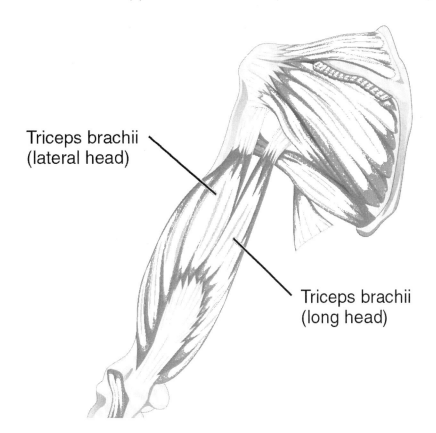

Triceps brachii (lateral head)

Triceps brachii (long head)

Left upper arm muscles (posterior view)

The forearm is extended by increasing the angle at the elbow and extending the hand away from the shoulder. The triceps brachii muscle is principally responsible for this movement. Extensor muscles located in the posterior compartment of the forearm (also known as the extensor compartment), such as the extensor carpi radialis longus, extensor carpi radialis brevis, extensor digitorum, extensor carpi ulnaris, and anconeus, also contribute to forearm extension. These muscles only play a minimal role in forearm extension.

## 4.5 THE WRIST

Wrist flexion is the movement of the wrist to pull the palm of the hand downward. Several muscles, including the flexor carpi radialis, flexor carpi ulnaris, flexor digitorum superficialis, flexor digitorum profundus, and flexor pollicis longus, perform this activity.

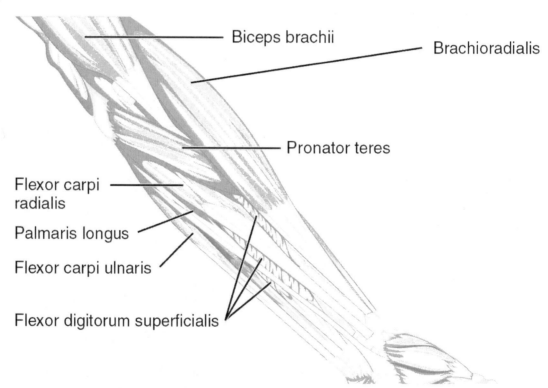

Left forearm superficial muscles (palmar view)

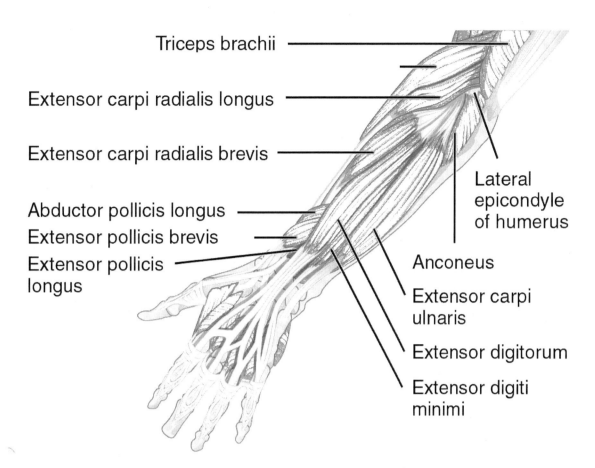

Triceps brachii

Extensor carpi radialis longus

Extensor carpi radialis brevis

Abductor pollicis longus
Extensor pollicis brevis
Extensor pollicis longus

Lateral epicondyle of humerus

Anconeus

Extensor carpi ulnaris

Extensor digitorum

Extensor digiti minimi

Left forearm superficial muscles (dorsal view)

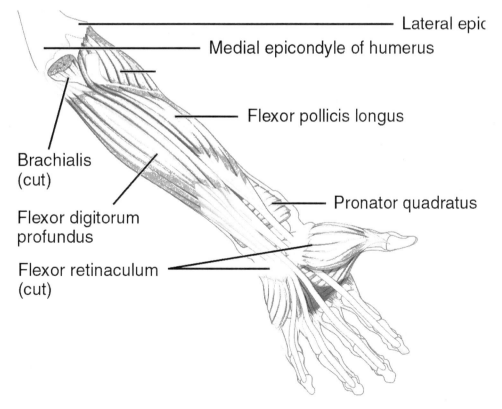

Lateral epic

Medial epicondyle of humerus

Flexor pollicis longus

Brachialis (cut)

Pronator quadratus

Flexor digitorum profundus

Flexor retinaculum (cut)

Left forearm deep muscles (palmar view)

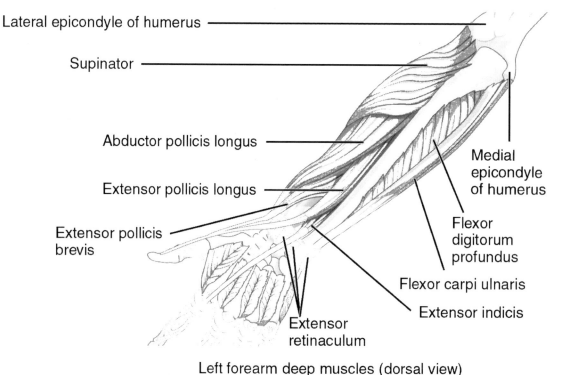

Lateral epicondyle of humerus

Supinator

Abductor pollicis longus

Extensor pollicis longus

Extensor pollicis brevis

Medial epicondyle of humerus

Flexor digitorum profundus

Flexor carpi ulnaris

Extensor indicis

Extensor retinaculum

Left forearm deep muscles (dorsal view)

Wrist extension, on the other hand, includes shortening the angle of the wrist at the rear. The extensor carpi radialis longus and brevis, which also abduct the hand at the wrist, the extensor digitorum, which also extends the index to little finger, the extensor digiti minimi, which also extends the little finger and adducts the hand, and the extensor carpi ulnaris, which also adducts the hand, are the muscles responsible for this action. Other minor muscles that straddle the wrist joint may also have a role in wrist extension, but to a lesser extent.

Wrist supination is the rotation of the wrist that causes the palm to face up, which is predominantly achieved by the supinator and biceps brachii muscles in the posterior compartment. The opposing movement is pronation, which involves rotating the wrist so that the palm faces down. The pronator quadratus, a deep muscle in the anterior compartment, and the pronator teres muscle perform this action.

## 4.6 The Abdomen

The abdominal wall is made up of three muscular layers, with a fourth layer in the midsection. The rectus abdominis is the fourth layer, with vertically oriented muscle fibers that flex the trunk and support the pelvis. The other three abdominal muscular layers are found on either side of the rectus abdominis. The transversus abdominis is the deepest layer, with fibers that run perpendicular to the rectus abdominis. The transversus abdominis compresses and supports the abdomen, allowing for static core stability.

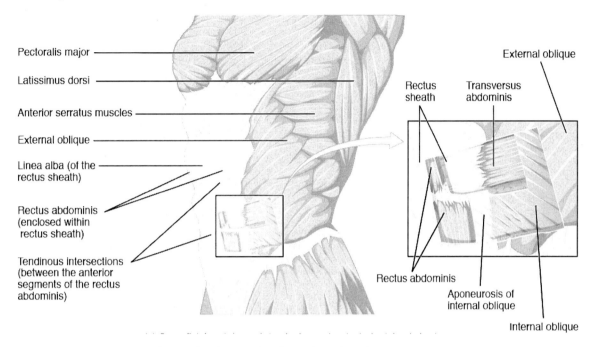

*OpenStax College - The abdominal wall muscles Wikimedia Commons CC BY 3.0*

Internal oblique muscles go upward and forward from the sides of the abdomen, whereas external oblique muscles flow downward and forward from the belly's outermost layer. The internal and external oblique muscles collaborate to flex and rotate the trunk to the side of the contracting internal oblique (also known as the "same-side rotator").

These muscles work together to keep the trunk stable and mobile, as well as to protect the abdominal organs. They are also useful in tasks involving the transmission of forces between the upper and lower bodies, such as tossing a ball or lifting a heavy object. These muscles may be strengthened to enhance core stability, posture, and athletic performance while lowering the risk of injury.

## 4.7  THE HIP

The hip joint is a weight-bearing, sophisticated ball-and-socket joint that can handle high stresses.

The joint's socket is somewhat deep, which provides stability but limits range of motion. Hip joint motions include flexion, extension, abduction, and adduction.

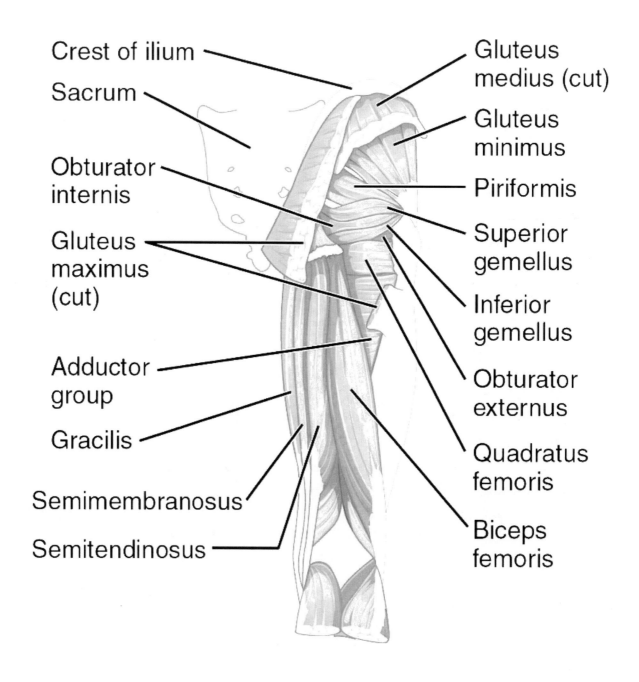

Crest of ilium

Sacrum

Obturator internis

Gluteus maximus (cut)

Adductor group

Gracilis

Semimembranosus

Semitendinosus

Gluteus medius (cut)

Gluteus minimus

Piriformis

Superior gemellus

Inferior gemellus

Obturator externus

Quadratus femoris

Biceps femoris

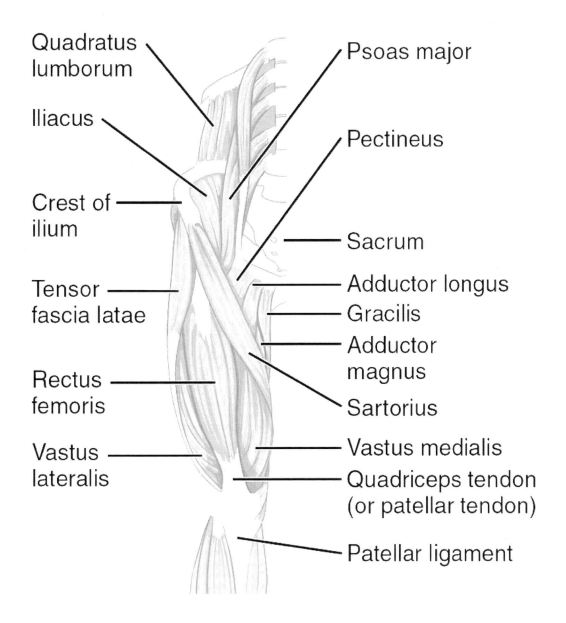

Quadratus lumborum

Iliacus

Crest of ilium

Tensor fascia latae

Rectus femoris

Vastus lateralis

Psoas major

Pectineus

Sacrum

Adductor longus

Gracilis

Adductor magnus

Sartorius

Vastus medialis

Quadriceps tendon (or patellar tendon)

Patellar ligament

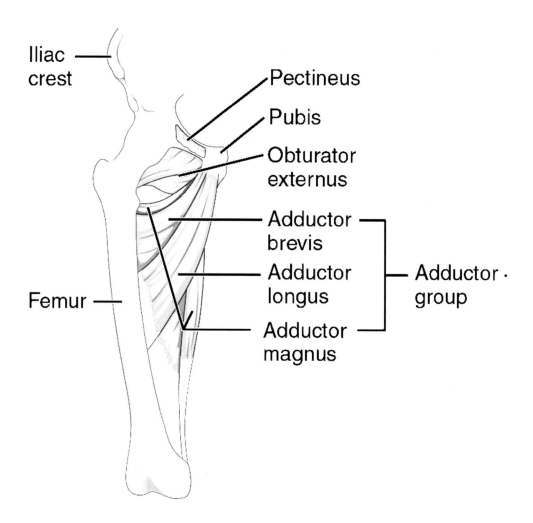

*OpenStax College - Human leg muscles Wikimedia Commons CC BY 3.0*

Hip flexion is the movement of bringing the knee up to the chest. The iliopsoas muscles, which consist of the psoas major, psoas minor, and iliacus muscles, are the primary muscles involved in hip flexion. These muscles predominantly flex the hip, although they also help with abdominal flexion and hip stability. The sartorius, rectus femoris, pectineus, and gracilis muscles are also hip flexors. The sartorius muscle also helps with external hip rotation, knee extension, and abduction, whereas the rectus femoris helps with knee extension. The pectineus muscle helps in hip adduction and internal rotation.

The muscles of the posterior thigh and buttocks are largely responsible for hip extension, which entails extending the thigh from a flexed position towards the midline of the body or from a bent position into an upright posture. The key muscles involved for hip extension are the gluteus maximus, biceps femoris (long and short heads), semitendinosus, and semimembranosus. This action is aided by the adductor magnus and other small pelvic muscles.

A limb is adducted when it moves toward the midline of the body. The gluteus medius, gluteus minimus, and tensor fascia lata are the primary abductors of the hip. These muscles also help in internal thigh rotation in an extended posture and external thigh rotation in a flexed position. The piriformis muscle only plays a modest role in hip abduction. The primary hip adductors are the adductor magnus, adductor brevis, and adductor longus, with the pectineus and gracilis muscles contributing just little to hip adduction.

## 4.8 THE THIGH AND UPPER LEG

The quadriceps femoris muscle group is primarily responsible for knee extension, which involves increasing the angle of the knee and straightening the lower leg. This movement is necessary for activities like walking and kicking. The vastus medialis, vastus lateralis, vastus intermedius, and rectus femoris muscles are all part of the quadriceps femoris group. The sartorius muscle also helps in knee extension, but to a lesser extent.

Knee flexion, on the other hand, is defined as the bending of the knee joint from a straight posture. The hamstring muscles, which are positioned at the back of the thigh and include the biceps femoris, semitendinosus, and semimembranosus, are responsible for this action. The gastrocnemius muscle at the rear of the calf and many minor muscles that cross the knee joint posteriorly contribute to knee flexion. Activities requiring knee flexion include running, leaping, and squatting.

## 4.9 THE FOOT AND LOWER LEG

Plantarflexion is ankle flexion in the direction of the plantar surface of the foot (the ground-contact surface of the foot). The gastrocnemius and soleus muscles, which compose the triceps surae muscle group, do plantarflexion. The gastrocnemius muscle is in charge of creating strong contractions, whereas the soleus muscle is in charge of maintaining upright position. Plantarflexion is also aided by the plantaris muscle, a tiny muscle found behind the knee.

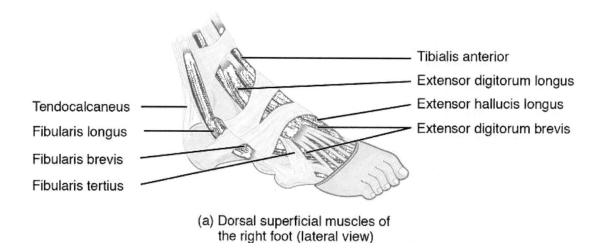

Tibialis anterior

Extensor digitorum longus

Extensor hallucis longus

Extensor digitorum brevis

Tendocalcaneus

Fibularis longus

Fibularis brevis

Fibularis tertius

(a) Dorsal superficial muscles of
the right foot (lateral view)

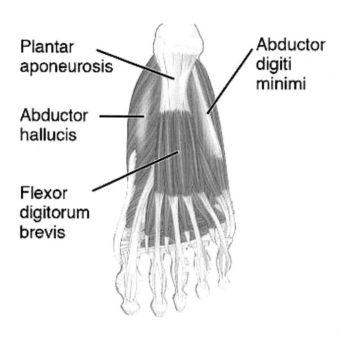

Plantar
aponeurosis

Abductor
digiti
minimi

Abductor
hallucis

Flexor
digitorum
brevis

(b) Superficial muscles of the
left sole (plantar view)

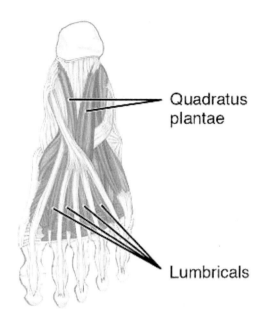

(c) Intermediate muscles of
the left sole (plantar view)

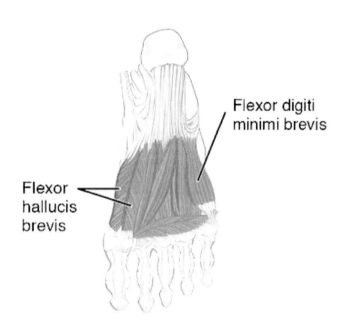

(d) Deep muscles of the
left sole (plantar view)

*OpenStax- The human foot's muscles, tendons, and nerves Wikimedia Commons CC BY 4.0*

The motions of the foot in the frontal plane are referred to as inversion and eversion. Inversion entails raising the medial (inner) edge of the foot while lowering the lateral (outer) edge, whereas eversion involves raising the lateral edge while lowering the medial edge. The tibialis anterior, tibialis posterior, and flexor digitorum longus muscles are responsible for inversion. The peroneus longus, peroneus brevis, and peroneus tertius muscles are responsible for eversion.

Lower leg and foot muscles are essential for balance, walking, running, and other weight-bearing movements. Exercise can help to strengthen these muscles, which can enhance sports performance and lessen the chance of injury.

Plantarflexion is an ankle joint action that involves flexion in the direction of the foot's sole. It's easiest to show by standing on one's toes. The gastrocnemius and soleus muscles, collectively known as the triceps surae, are the major muscles responsible for ankle plantarflexion. Plantarflexion is also aided to a lesser amount by the plantaris muscle, which runs obliquely between the gastrocnemius and the soleus.

The flexor hallucis longus, which primarily contributes to big toe flexion but also aids in ankle plantarflexion; the flexor digitorum longus, which flexes the second to fifth toes and also aids in ankle plantarflexion; the peroneus longus, which flexes the ankle and everts the foot; and the peroneus brevis, which contributes to ankle plantarflexion and foot eversion. These muscles are required for balance, walking, and other weight-bearing tasks.

The intrinsic muscles of the foot are fully contained inside the foot and are responsible for numerous toe motions. The big toe is abducted by the abductor hallucis muscle, whereas the second to fifth toes are flexed by the flexor digitorum brevis muscle. The fifth toe is abducted and flexed by the abductor digiti minimi muscle, and toe flexion is assisted by the quadratus plantae muscle.

The lumbrical muscles are responsible for flexing the metatarsophalangeal joints as well as extending the distal and proximal interphalangeal joints of the toes. The flexor hallucis brevis muscle flexes the big toe, whereas the adductor hallucis muscle contracts it. The adductor hallucis muscle has two heads: the oblique head, which originates from the base of the second to fourth metatarsal bones, and the transverse head, which originates from the ligaments of the third to fifth metatarsophalangeal joints.

The flexor digiti minimi brevis muscle extends and adducts the fifth toe, whereas the dorsal and plantar interossei muscles abduct and adduct the toes. These muscles collaborate to give foot stability and control during actions such as walking, running, and jumping.

# Conclusion

To summarize, the human body is an extraordinarily complicated and interesting mechanism, with each component critical to our general health and well-being. We've looked at the several systems that make up the human body, from the skeletal system to the muscular system. We've studied about the many architecture and functions of each system, as well as how they all work together to keep our bodies running smoothly.

We can better appreciate the intricacy of our bodies and the importance of taking care of them if we have a greater understanding of human anatomy. Whether you are a student, a healthcare professional, or simply someone who enjoys learning, this book has given you a thorough introduction to the fascinating world of human anatomy.

We would like to thank Wikimedia and Britannica in particular for being helpful resources in the preparation of this book. Their huge databases of photographs and information enabled us to present a full introduction to human anatomy, for which we are grateful.

Finally, as you conclude this book, we hope you have gained a greater respect for the complexities and beauty of the human body. We encourage you to keep learning and exploring this fascinating topic, as well as to utilize what you have learned to improve your own health and well-being. Thank you for coming along on this adventure of discovery with us, and we wish you the best of luck in your future pursuits.

Made in United States
North Haven, CT
15 September 2023